Terrorism Emergency Response

A Workbook for Responders

Gordon M. Sachs

Prentice Hall
Upper Saddle River, New Jersey 07458

Library of Congress Cataloging-in-Publication Data
Sachs, Gordon M.
Terrorism emergency response : a workbook for responders / Gordon M. Sachs.
p. cm.
At head of title: Brady.
Includes bibliographical references and index.
ISBN 0-13-099364-6
1. Terrorism. 2. Medical emergencies. 3. Emergency medical technicians.
I. Title.

RC88.9.T47 S23 2002
616.02'5—dc21 2002028533

Note: Emergency personnel are reminded that they are required to comply with local response protocols as established within the jurisdiction that they are rendering service.

Publisher: *Julie Levin Alexander*
Publisher's Assistant: *Regina Bruno*
Senior Acquisitions Editor: *Katrin Beacom*
Editorial Assistant: *Kierra Kashickey*
Senior Marketing Manager: *Tiffany Price/Katrin Beacom*
Product Information Manager: *Rachele Strober*
Director of Production and Manufacturing: *Bruce Johnson*
Managing Production Editor: *Patrick Walsh*
Manufacturing Buyer: *Pat Brown*
Production Liaison: *Julie Li*
Production Editor: *Judith Schaeffer, Stratford Publishing Services*
Creative Director: *Cheryl Asherman*
Cover Design Coordinator: *Christopher Weigand*
Cover Designer: *Kevin Kall*
Compositor: *Stratford Publishing Services*
Printer/Binder: *R. R. Donnelley & Sons*
Cover Printer: *Phoenix Color Corporation*

Pearson Education LTD.
Pearson Education Australia PTY, Limited
Pearson Education Singapore, Pte. Ltd.
Pearson Education North Asia Ltd.
Pearson Education Canada, Ltd.
Pearson Educación de Mexico, S.A. de C.V.
Pearson Education—Japan
Pearson Education Malaysia, Pte. Ltd.
Pearson Education, Upper Saddle River, New Jersey

Prentice Hall

10 9 8 7 6 5 3 2
ISBN 0-13-099364-6

Contents

Dedication and Acknowledgments

This book is dedicated to all of the emergency responders around the world who have been injured or have died as a result of terrorist acts, and especially those fire, EMS, and law enforcement personnel who were killed or injured due to the attacks on September 11, 2001.

Thanks go to David Marron, Braddock Heights (MD) Fire Department; Eric Nagle, Cashtown (PA) Fire Company; Steve Weissman, Fairfax County (VA) Fire & Rescue Department; David Millstein, William Morton, and Lisa Sachs, Fairfield (PA) Fire & EMS; and Retsy Adelsberger, IOCAD Emergency Services Group, for their assistance in developing the scenarios for this workbook. Thanks also go to the course developers and instructors of the National Fire Academy's *Emergency Response to Terrorism* curriculum and to the staff of the U.S. Fire Administration's Response Branch for working so diligently to protect America's emergency responders from the perils of terrorism through training, research, and support.

Introduction

Because of the complex and myriad factors involved, terrorism is and will remain a dynamic topic. As terrorist-related incidents occur within the United States and around the world, effective methods of response to those incidents will be developed, studied, reviewed, and incorporated by response organizations. It will be important for all emergency response agencies to evaluate the lessons learned and formulate protocols for local emergency response to terrorism. This evaluation process must continue as other terrorist-related incidents occur, both domestically and internationally, in order to ensure that the necessary changes are made in response methodology.

In general, as the twentieth century progressed, terrorism increased. As we all know, a huge jump in the awareness, visibility, and impact of terrorism in the United States occurred at the beginning of the twenty-first century. A decade-by-decade examination of the number of terrorist incidents indicates an overall upward trend. For emergency responders, this raises two important considerations. First, they are being called upon to respond to an increasing number of terrorist-related incidents. Recent events within the United States clearly indicate that these incidents can and will take place on the "home front," and the potential is great that they will continue. Second, emergency services personnel in fire, EMS, and law enforcement must seriously consider the fact that they themselves may well be the targets of terrorist aggression.

The first instinct for emergency responders at any incident is always to rush in and save as many people as possible; however, in a terrorist-related incident there are many factors to consider. Can the victims be saved? Will responders become targets? Was an agent of some type released? If it was, will responders have the means to detect it? Will their gear provide adequate protection? These are but a few of the questions that we must become accustomed to asking when responding to terrorist-related incidents. There is no reason to allow civilians to suffer needlessly; neither can there be any reason to send responders haphazardly into unknown and dangerous environments. Responding to acts of terrorism means facing many unfortunate realities. The decisions made by the incident commander during responses to these acts are therefore more critical than ever before.

The intent of this workbook is to reinforce basic information about types of terrorist incidents that emergency response personnel—fire, rescue, EMS, haz-mat, law enforcement—may face and to provide scenarios that any of these responders can use to help sharpen the decision-making skills needed if encountering a terrorist event. The main thrust is to help keep the responder from becoming a victim.

About the Author

Gordon M. Sachs has over twenty-five years of fire service and EMS experience, including more than ten years as a chief officer in both career and volunteer departments. Currently, he is chief of Fairfield Fire and EMS in Pennsylvania and is the director of the IOCAD Emergency Services Group, a consulting firm providing management and technical support for FEMA, the U.S. Fire Administration, the National Fire Academy, and emergency services across the country. He holds a Master of Public Administration degree and a Bachelor of Science in education, and is a graduate of the National Fire Academy's Executive Fire Officer program. Chief Sachs is the author of *Officer's Guide to Fire Service EMS* (Fire Engineering Books, 1999) and *Fire & EMS Department Safety Officer* (Brady, 2000). He has coauthored several books and publications, including *Fire Department Occupational Health and Safety Handbook* (NFPA, 1998) and *The Fire Chief's Handbook, Fifth Edition* and *Sixth Edition* (Fire Engineering Books, 1995 and 2002), as well as several U.S. Fire Administration publications. He has also written numerous trade journal articles and made several major presentations in the areas of fire service/EMS leadership and management, emergency responder health and safety, incident command, and emergency response to terrorism. Chief Sachs is a course developer and adjunct instructor at the National Fire Academy and is a guest lecturer at several colleges and universities. He is a former U.S. Fire Administration Program manager and has been a member of several national committees, including NFPA technical committees and various federal and state committees on emergency service issues.

1 History of the Use of Chemical, Biological, and Radiological Agents

CHEMICAL AGENTS

423 B.C.	Allies of Sparta in the Peloponnesian War took an Athenian-held fort by directing smoke from lighted coals, sulfur, and pitch through a hollowed-out beam into the fort.
7th century A.D.	Greeks invented "Greek Fire"—a combination of rosin, sulfur, pitch, naphtha, lime, and saltpeter. This floated on the water and was particularly effective in naval operations.
19th century A.D.	Nineteenth-century proposals that were never put into practice included using chlorine-filled shells against the Confederacy during the American Civil War and dipping bayonets into cyanide (the suggestion of Napoleon III during the Franco-Prussian War).
1915	German units released an estimated 150 tons of chlorine gas from some 6,000 cylinders near Ypres, Belgium. Although this attack caused only 800 deaths, it was psychologically devastating to the 15,000 Allied troops, who promptly retreated.
1917	German artillery shells delivered a new kind of chemical agent, sulfur mustard, causing 20,000 casualties.
Post-WWI	Chemicals were allegedly used against Russians and mustard against the Afghans north of the Khyber Pass. Spain is said to have employed mustard shells and bombs

	against the Riff tribes of Morocco. During the next decade, the Soviet Union supposedly used lung irritants against tribesmen in Kurdistan.
1936	Mussolini, who used tear gas during the war against Abyssinia, also authorized massive aerial delivery of mustard against Abyssinian tribesmen and as an interdiction movement on Italian flanks.
WWII	Germany weaponized thousands of tons of organophosphates, which came to be called nerve agents. However, they were never used during the war.
1980	Widely publicized reports of Iraqi use of chemical agents against Iran during the 1980s led to a U.N. investigation that confirmed the use of the vesicant mustard and the nerve agent tabun (GA). Later during the war, Iraq apparently also began to use the more volatile nerve agent sarin (GB), and Iran may have used chemical agents to a limited extent in an attempt to retaliate for Iraqi attacks. Press reports also implicated cyanide in the deaths of Kurds.

BIOLOGICAL AGENTS

6th century B.C	Assyrians poisoned enemy wells with rye ergot. Solon of Athens used the purgative herb hellebore to poison the water supply during the siege of Krissa.
1346	Plague broke out in the Tartar army during its siege of Kaffa. The attackers hurled the corpses of those who died over the city walls. Although it is most likely the disease spread in the city by rats rather than from the enemy corpses, the plague epidemic that followed forced the defenders to surrender, and some infected people who left

Kaffa may have started the Black Death pandemic, which spread throughout Europe.

1763 Captain Simeon Ecuyer, a British officer under the command of General Sir Jeffrey Amherst, distributed smallpox-infected blankets to Indians during the French and Indian War in North America.

1797 Napoleon attempted to infect the inhabitants of the besieged city of Mantua with swamp fever during his Italian campaign.

1915 Dr. Anton Dilger established a small biological agent production facility at his Washington, DC home. Using cultures of anthrax and glanders, Dilger produced an estimated liter of liquid agent. The agent and a simple inoculation device were given to a group of dock workers in Baltimore, who used them to infect 3,000 head of horses, mules, and cattle destined for the Allied forces in Europe.

1931 Japanese military officials tried to poison members of the League of Nations' Lytton Commission, assigned to investigate Japan's seizure of Manchuria in 1931, by lacing fruit with cholera bacteria.

1939–1945 Japanese established a biological weapons program, known as Unit 731, at Ping Fan, Manchuria, and other cities in China. Human experiments were conducted and 3,000 prisoners died.

1972 In Chicago, members of a U.S. right-wing group known as the "Order of the Rising Sun" were arrested. The group was dedicated to creating a new master race and possessed 30 to 40 kilograms of typhoid bacteria cultures for use against water supplies in Chicago, St. Louis, and other Midwestern cities.

1978/1979	In 1978, Bulgarian agents assassinated Georgi Markov in London using a ricin pellet and attempted to assassinate Vladimir Kostov. In 1979, an accident happened at a secretive military base called "Compound 19." Behind walls, a deadly production line turned out tons of anthrax powder for the Soviet Union's biological arsenal. One April morning, a small amount of the dust was accidentally released through the ventilation system. The invisible plume was blown over a working-class neighborhood and nearby ceramics factory, killing between sixty and eighty people.
1983	The FBI arrested two brothers in the northeastern United States who had manufactured an ounce of nearly pure ricin, stored in a 35-mm film canister.
1984	One bioterrorism incident in the United States occurred in September 1984 and involved the Rajneeshee, a religious cult, which had established a large commune in Wasco County east of Portland, Oregon. Relations between the county's residents and the cult had been extremely contentious, leading the cult to adopt a plan to take over the county by manipulating the results of the November 1984 election. They planned to bus homeless people into their commune and register them as voters, while at the same time making the opposing voters sick and thus unable to vote on election day. To sicken the voters of Wasco County, the cult grew *Salmonella typhimurium*, which causes a diarrheal disease, from a culture purchased from a medical supply house. To test their new weapon, the cult tried unsuccessfully to spread the disease during August 1984 in the county

seat. On August 29th, they gave water laced with *S. typhimurium* to two county commissioners the Rajneeshee considered hostile. Both became sick; one required hospitalization. Although the Rajneeshee were suspected of deliberately poisoning the commissioners, there was no evidence to support such a claim and there was no criminal investigation. In September 1984, the Rajneeshees redoubled their efforts by contaminating the salad bars of ten restaurants. They spread the disease by pouring vials of media containing the organism over the foods. The result was an estimated 751 cases of salmonellosis. However, the actual number could have been higher, because the community is on an interstate and some of the infected travelers may not have reported their illness. Also in 1984, in Paris, a Red Army faction "safe house" was discovered that contained a primitive laboratory containing cultures of *Clostridium botulinum*. Botulinum toxin is one of the most toxic substances known.

1995 On March 15, 1995, the Aum Shinrikyo placed three briefcases designed to release botulinum toxin in the Tokyo subway. Apparently, the individual responsible for filling the botulinum toxin had qualms about the planned attack and substituted a nontoxic substance. The failure of this attack led the cult to use sarin in its March 20, 1995, subway attack. The Aum Shinrikyo also used anthrax unsuccessfully.

RADIOLOGICAL AGENTS

1941 The use of radioactive materials as weapons was first considered during World War II.

The National Academy of Sciences proposed radiological warfare as a military application of atomic energy. In its report, the Academy's first option was the "production of violently radioactive materials carried by airplanes to be scattered as bombs over enemy territory." After British physicists demonstrated the technical feasibility of nuclear explosive weapons, attention quickly turned to their development throughout the remainder of the war.

1946 The United States conducted the Operation Crossroads nuclear weapons tests at Bikini Atoll in the Marshall Islands. The widespread contamination of ships used in these tests dramatically proved the potential of radiological warfare.

1947 The Defense Department began studying the offensive and defensive aspects of "Rad War." This led to an active test program that included releases of radiation into the atmosphere in the 1940s and 1950s. These early experiments showed that while radiological devices were not effective as battlefield weapons, such weapons could have a significant psychological effect. Yet, for the next four decades, there was little documented interest in developing radiological weapons. With the advent of global terrorism, this option has again drawn attention.

2 Safe Operations at Terrorist Incidents

TERRORISM DEFINED

Terrorism is defined by the federal government as "the use of force or violence against persons or property to intimidate or coerce a government, the civilian population, or any segment thereof to further political or social objectives." Terrorists have the knowledge and capability to strike anywhere in the world, and will do whatever they believe they have to do to achieve their goal. They have shown that they will use weapons of mass destruction (WMD) without hesitation.

In recent years we have seen an increasing number of attacks in the United States against the government and civilians from both foreign and domestic groups. These include:

- Jonesboro, AK—Armed attack at school
- Oregon—Biological agent dispersed in restaurant salad bars
- Atlanta, GA—Olympics bombing
- Atlanta, GA—Abortion clinic bombing, night club bombing
- Littleton, CO—Armed attack at school
- Vail, CO—Incendiary attack (arson) at ski resort
- Fairfax, VA—CIA armed attack
- New York City, NY—World Trade Center bombing
- Oklahoma City, OK—Federal building bombing
- Palm Beach County, FL—Anthrax attacks
- Washington, DC, and New York City, NY—Anthrax attacks via mail
- New York City, NY; Arlington, VA; and Shanksville, PA—Attacks using hijacked airplanes

Terrorism took on a new dimension in the minds of Americans after the September 11, 2001, attacks on the World Trade Center and the Pentagon. We no longer view our vulnerability in terms of isolated incidents. Our concept of terrorist tactics has changed forever. We now think of airplanes used for routine domestic flights as possible weapons. The bioterrorist threat became a reality with the spread of anthrax through the U.S. Postal Service. The concern exists that even emergency response vehicles can become weapons. Moreover, we know that responders themselves can be targets. Recent events have shown that a carefully timed sequence of events may be planned to inflict further harm to those who respond to the initial incident. These events may include:

- Armed resistance
- Use of weapons
- Booby traps
- Secondary events

CATEGORIES OF TERRORIST INCIDENTS

Biological Incidents

Biological agents are fairly accessible and rapidly spread. Biological agents include anthrax, tularemia, cholera, plague, botulism, and smallpox. These agents can be distributed in a variety of ways: inhalation (aerosol spray or fine powder), ingestion (food or water contamination), direct skin contact, or injection.

Nuclear Incidents

There are two types of nuclear threats. The first is the threatened detonation of a nuclear bomb. The second is the threatened or actual detonation of a conventional explosive incorporating nuclear material. Although the potential for a terrorist organization to gain nuclear devices has been considered minimal, with the recent changes in terrorist events it is possible and has became a significant threat.

Incendiary Incidents

An incendiary device is any mechanical, electrical, or chemical device used intentionally to initiate combustion and start a fire. Incendiary devices may be simple or complex and come in all shapes and sizes. The type of device is limited only by the terrorist's imagination and ingenuity. Only specially trained personnel should handle incendiary devices discovered prior to ignition.

Chemical Incidents

Chemical agents fall into five classes:

- Nerve agents
- Vesicant agents (formerly known as blister agents)
- Cyanogens (formerly known as blood agents)
- Pulmonary agents (formerly known as choking agents)
- Riot control agents (also known as irritating agents)

The primary routes of exposure to chemical agents are inhalation, ingestion, and skin absorption.

Explosive Incidents

It is estimated that 70 percent of worldwide terrorist attacks involve explosives. Bombings are the most likely terrorist attack to be encountered. Explosions rapidly release gas and heat, affecting both people and structures. Bombs almost always work as designed; few misfire or are "duds." It is important to remember that explosions can cause fires and fires can cause explosions. Responders must always be aware of the potential for secondary devices.

POTENTIAL RESPONDER INJURIES

There are many possible sources of injuries to firefighters and other emergency personnel responding to a terrorist incident. These include:

- Improvised explosive devices
- Secondary explosive devices
- Firearms
- Exposure to chemicals
- Trapped and injured in building collapse
- Exposure to biological agents
- Exposure to infectious diseases
- Burns from incendiary fire
- Injuries due to debris from explosion or collapse of building
- Overexertion

There are no easy ways to protect responders from these dangers, but self-protection is built on the three key areas used for hazardous materials incidents: time, distance, and shielding.

Time: You should spend the shortest amount of time possible in the hazard area. Use techniques such as rapid entries to conduct reconnaissance and rescue. Minimizing time spent in the affected area also reduces the chance of contaminating the crime scene.

Distance: It should be an absolute rule to maintain a safe distance from the hazard area or projected hazard area. If at all possible, be upwind and uphill from the source. An excellent resource for determining safe distances is the Table of Initial Isolation and Protective Action Distances found in the *North American Emergency Response Guidebook*. This book is typically carried on all emergency response vehicles; additional copies are available through local and state emergency management agencies.

Shielding: Shields can take various forms, such as vehicles, buildings, walls, and personal protective equipment (PPE). However, no matter how much shielding is available, always take full advantage of time and distance.

INCIDENT RESPONSE CONSIDERATIONS

Clues

Responders must look for clues that will indicate that an incident involves terrorism. These clues include:

- Type of occupancy—High occupancy, politically sensitive services such as abortion clinics
- Type of event—Political rally, for example
- Type of incident—Explosion, for example
- Type of incident combined with time of day
- Dead animals or insects in area
- Type of incident combined with occupancy factor
- Historic dates—anniversary of a previous attack, for example
- Vapor clouds
- Unexplained containers
- Victims with abnormal injuries—numerous people having seizures, for example

The United States Fire Administration publishes the *Emergency Response to Terrorism: Job Aid*, which is designed to assist the first responder from the fire, EMS, haz-mat, and law enforcement disciplines in identifying a possible terrorist/WMD incident and implementing initial actions. This document is not a training manual but a "memory jogger" for those who have completed the appropriate level of training. This publication is available to emergency response organizations only and can be ordered online from USFA Publications at http://www.usfa.fema.gov.

First-In Officer

The first-in officer should approach the scene upwind and upgrade if possible to avoid exposure to any potential hazardous materials. The old adage, "Fools rush in where angels fear to tread," is well worth remembering. Assessing the scene using binoculars and gathering information from citizens and/or other government personnel who have left the immediate are can be a lifesaver for the responders who are about to enter. Other responding units should be assigned positions in locations that provide a multidimensional view of the scene. Monitoring devices should be employed and all personnel should wear appropriate personal protective equipment.

Additional measures should be employed if the incident involves an armed attack. Personnel should be protected with a hard barrier and remain mobile. It is essential to immediately establish communication with the law enforcement officials on the scene. This could be lifesaving to all responders. Mobile treatment areas for victims should be established in a safe place with hard cover and law enforcement support. Victims should not be removed from the area until it has been secured and is safe. A lookout should be assigned to watch for any changes in the scene that would indicate immediate or increasing danger.

Initial Operations Team

An initial operations team should conduct the initial risk assessment of the area and should be composed of six to ten personnel with a variety of special training. The team should include the following specialties:

- Hazardous materials
- Law enforcement
- Monitoring
- Advanced life support
- Forcible entry/victim removal personnel and equipment

The initial operations team may enter the incident area only when it is determined that the area is safe. The strategic goals of the team are general, such as:

- Provide safe operations for all public safety personnel
- Identify and, if feasible, rescue/evacuate viable victims
- Confine incident, loss of life, and damage to area of origin

Because this team is multiagency, the line of authority must be clear so the team functions in an organized, mission-driven approach. Before entering the area, an emergency evacuation signal, escape routes, and rallying points must be established. There should be two backup teams and one cover team (as required) in place. The team must make a cautious, deliberate approach to the area from upwind and upgrade. Once in the area, the team will:

- Determine the source (blast, chemical, etc.)
- Determine risks versus benefits

  (Low gain/high risk—no)

  (Moderate gain/low risk—go)

  (Low gain/moderate risk—no)

  (High gain/low risk—go)
- Identify/establish operational zones
- Identify proper PPE needed by subsequent entry teams
- Report the situation and resource status to the incident commander

The incident commander will order withdrawal or support based on the report received from the initial operations team.

SAFETY OPERATIONS

Safety for these types of incidents also requires a team approach. The team should consist of the incident safety officer, law enforcement, technical advisors, assistant safety officers, and special operational personnel (government and private). The safety operations team must also communicate closely with the incident commander (to evaluate and establish operational zones) and emergency medical services (to review exposure symptoms and treatment protocols). Other responsibilities include:

- Reviewing, updating, and communicating escape routes regularly
- Establishing exposure and documentation procedures

- Notifying medical facilities of the situation for the safety of their staff
- Monitoring weather and its impact on operations
- Monitoring time on scene
- Reviewing Rapid Intervention Crew operations
- Reviewing staging locations and procedures
- Reviewing staffing and location of law enforcement
- Reviewing site restriction protocols, procedures, and effectiveness
- Providing rehabilitation areas

3 Effects of Biological, Chemical, and Radiological Agents

Experts generally agree that there are five categories of terrorist incidents: biological, nuclear, incendiary, chemical, and explosive. The acronym *B-NICE* is a simple way to remember the five categories.

BIOLOGICAL AGENTS

Biological agents pose very serious threats given their accessibility and their ability to spread rapidly. The potential for devastating casualties is high in a biological incident. These agents are disseminated in the following ways: inhalation (by the use of aerosols), ingestion (contaminating food or water supplies), dermal exposure (direct skin contact with the substance), or injection (which is unlikely in a terrorist situation).

There are four common types of biological agents: bacteria, rickettsia, viruses, and toxins. The primary routes of exposure for these agents are inhalation and ingestion. Skin absorption and injection are potential routes of entry, but are less likely.

Several biological agents can be adapted and used as terrorist weapons. These include anthrax (sometimes found in sheep), tularemia (or rabbit fever), cholera, encephalitis, the plague (sometimes found in prairie dog colonies), and botulism (found in improperly canned food).

Bacteria and Rickettsia

Bacteria are single-celled organisms that multiply by cell division and can cause disease in humans, plants, or animals. Although true cells, rickettsia are smaller than bacteria and live inside individual host cells. Examples of bacteria include anthrax (*Bacillus anthracis*), cholera (*Vibrio cholerae*), plague (*Yersinia pestis*), and tularemia (*Francisella tularensis*). An example of rickettsia is Q fever (*Coxiella burnetii*).

You may be familiar with the disease anthrax, which is associated with cattle, sheep, and horses as hosts. Handling of contaminated hair, wool, hides, flesh, or other animal substances can lead to contracting cutaneous (dermal) anthrax. However, the purposeful dissemination of spores in aerosol, such as for terrorist purposes, could also spread contamination and cause a more dangerous form of the disease.

Viruses

Viruses are the simplest type of microorganisms. They lack a system for their own metabolism and therefore depend upon living cells to multiply. This means that a virus will not live long outside of a host.

Types of viruses that could serve as biological agents include smallpox, Venezuelan equine encephalitis, and the viral hemorrhagic fevers, such as the Ebola and Marburg viruses and Lassa fever.

Toxins

Toxins are toxic substances of natural origin produced by an animal, plant, or microbe. They differ from chemical agents in that they are not manufactured and typically they are much more complex materials; however, biotoxins and chemical agents are more similar than different. Several toxins are easily extracted for use as a terrorist weapon and, by weight, usually are more toxic than many chemical agents.

The four common toxins thought of as potential biological agents are botulism (botulinum), SEB (staphylococcal enterotoxin B), ricin, and mycotoxins.

Ricin is a toxin derived from the castor bean plant, which is available worldwide. Terror groups and miscreants have published recipes for making ricin. There have been several documented cases involving ricin throughout the United States, particularly in rural areas.

NUCLEAR INCIDENTS

There are two fundamentally different threats in the area of nuclear terrorism. One is the use, threatened use, or threatened detonation of a nuclear bomb. The other is the detonation, or threatened detonation, of a conventional explosive device incorporating nuclear materials (radiological dispersal devices, or RDD).

Nuclear Bomb Threats

It is unlikely that any terrorist organization could acquire or build a nuclear device, or acquire and use a fully functional nuclear weapon. The number of nations with nuclear capability is small, and each places a high priority on the control of its nuclear weapons. Even if a nation supporting terrorism could develop a nuclear capability, experts believe it would be implausible for that nation to turn a completed weapon over to a group that might use it against them.

The theft of a completed nuclear weapon also is unlikely. All nuclear nations have placed their nuclear arsenals under the highest security. All Western and former Soviet nuclear weapons are protected with a Permissible Action Link (PAL) system that renders the weapon harmless until the proper code is entered.

The greatest potential terrorist threat for a nuclear weapon would be to use such a device as a form of extortion. The U.S. government has plans to meet such a threatened use. Currently, there is no known nongovernment group close to obtaining or producing a nuclear weapon.

Nuclear Materials Threats

The purpose of an attack where nuclear materials are incorporated into a conventional explosive (RDD) would be to spread radioactive materials around the bomb site. This would disrupt normal, everyday activities, and would raise the level of concern among first responders regarding long-term health issues. It would be difficult to perform complete environmental decontamination.

Another possible scenario involving nuclear materials would be the detonation of a large device, such as a truck bomb (large vehicle with high quantities of explosives), in the vicinity of a nuclear power plant or a radiological cargo in transport. Such an attack could have widespread effects. The frequency of shipments of radiological materials is increasing throughout the world.

Radioactive materials emit three main types of nuclear radiation: alpha, beta, and gamma radiation.

Alpha: Alpha particles are the heaviest and most highly charged of the nuclear particles. However, alpha particles cannot travel more than a few inches in air and are completely stopped by an ordinary sheet of paper. The outermost layer of dead skin that covers the body can stop even the most energetic alpha particle. However, if ingested through eating, drinking, or breathing contaminated materials, they can become an internal hazard.

Beta: Beta particles are smaller and travel much faster than alpha particles. Typical beta particles can travel several millimeters through tissue, but they generally do not penetrate far enough to reach the vital inner organs. Exposure to beta particles from outside the body is normally thought of as a slight hazard. However, if the skin is exposed to large amounts of beta radiation for long periods of time, skin burns may result. If removed from the skin shortly after exposure, beta-emitting materials will not cause serious burns. Like alpha particles, beta particles are considered to be an internal hazard if taken into the body by eating, drinking, or breathing contaminated materials. Beta-emitting contamination can also enter the body through unprotected open wounds.

Gamma: Gamma rays are a type of electromagnetic radiation transmitted through space in the form of waves. Gamma rays are pure energy and therefore are the most penetrating type of radiation. They can travel great distances and can penetrate most materials. This creates a problem for humans, because gamma rays can attack all tissues and organs. Gamma radiation has very distinctive, short-term symptoms. Acute radiation sickness occurs when an individual is exposed to a large amount of radiation within a short period of time. Symptoms of acute radiation sickness include skin irritation, nausea, vomiting, high fever, hair loss, and dermal burns.

INCENDIARY INCIDENTS

An incendiary device is any mechanical, electrical, or chemical device used intentionally to initiate combustion and start a fire. A delay mechanism consists of chemical, electrical, or mechanical elements. These elements may be used singly or in combinations. Incendiary materials burn with a hot flame for a designated period of time. Their purpose is to set fire to other materials or structures.

Incendiary devices may be simple or elaborate and come in all shapes and sizes. The type of device is limited only by the terrorist's imagination and ingenuity. An incendiary device can be a simple match applied to a piece of paper, a matchbook-and-cigarette combination, or a complicated self-igniting chemical device. Normally, an incendiary device is a material or mixture of materials designed to produce enough heat and flame to cause combustible material to burn once it reaches its ignition temperature. Each device consists of three basic components: an igniter or fuse, a container or body, and an incendiary material or filler. The container can be glass, metal, plastic, or paper, depending on its desired use. A device containing chemical materials usually will be in a metal or other unbreakable container. An incendiary device that uses a liquid accelerator usually will be in a breakable container, such as glass. Generally, crime scene investigators find three types of incendiary devices: electrical, mechanical, or chemical. These may be used singularly or in combinations.

As with all WMD devices, only specially trained personnel should handle incendiary devices discovered prior to ignition. Handling of such devices by inexperienced individuals can result in ignition and possible injury or death. In addition, proper handling is critical for crime scene preservation.

The effects of incendiary agents are no different from those found in traditional responses. The skin is the primary organ involved, initially reddening and becoming painful (first degree burn). With more serious burns, the skin blisters and swells (second degree burn), and extremely serious burns can destroy all skin layers and result in charred, painless areas (third degree or full-thickness burn). Other systems that can be affected by burns include the respiratory tract, lungs, and eyes. Respiratory tract burns can be life-threatening due to swelling and resultant obstruction of the airway.

CHEMICAL AGENTS

Chemical agents fall into five classes: Nerve agents, which disrupt nerve impulse transmissions; vesicant agents, formerly called blister agents, which cause severe burns to eyes, skin, and tissues of the respiratory tract; cyanogens, which interfere with the ability of blood to transport oxygen; pulmonary agents, formerly called choking agents, which severely stress respiratory system tissues; and riot control agents, which can be either irritating agents or psychedelic (incapacitating) agents. Irritating agents cause respiratory distress and tearing, and can cause intense pain to the skin, especially in moist areas of the body. Psychedelic agents alter the nervous system and cause hallucinations and changes in thought processes and behavior.

The primary routes of exposure for chemical agents are inhalation, ingestion, and skin absorption or contact. Injection is a potential source of entry, but is less likely. With the exception of blister agents, inhalation is the primary route of exposure for chemical agents. However, skin absorption or contact with irritant nerve agents and blister agents also is a highly possible route of exposure.

Nerve Agents

Nerve agents are similar in nature to organophosphate pesticides, but with a higher degree of toxicity. All are toxic at small concentrations (a small drop could be fatal). The agents include sarin (GB), used by terrorists against Japanese civilians and by the Iraqis against Iran; soman (GD); tabun (GA); and V agent (VX). These materials are liquids that typically are disseminated by aerosol spray. In the case of GA, GB, and GD, the first letter "G" refers to the country (Germany) that developed the agent, and the second letter indicates the order of development. In the case of VX, the "V" stands for "venom" while the "X" represents one of the chemicals in the specific compound.

The victims' symptoms are an early outward warning sign of the use of nerve agents. There are various generic symptoms similar to organophosphate poisoning. The victims will salivate, lacrimate, urinate, and defecate without much control. Other symptoms may include:

- Eyes: Pinpointed pupils, dimmed and blurred vision, pain aggravated by sunlight
- Skin: Excessive sweating and fine muscle tremors
- Muscles: Involuntary twitching and contractions
- Respiratory system: Runny nose and nasal congestion, chest pressure and congestion, coughing and difficulty breathing
- Digestive system: Excessive salivation, abdominal pain, nausea and vomiting, involuntary defecation and urination
- Nervous system: Giddiness, anxiety, difficulty in thinking and sleeping (nightmares)

Nerve agents resemble water or light oil in pure form and possess no odor. The most efficient distribution is as an aerosol. Small explosions and equipment to generate mists (spray devices) may be present. Nerve agents kill insect life, birds, and other animals as well as humans. Many dead animals at the scene of an incident may be an outward warning sign or detection clue.

Vesicant Agents

Vesicants are also referred to as mustard agents due to their characteristic smell. They are similar to other corrosive materials first responders encounter. They readily penetrate layers of clothing and are quickly absorbed into the skin. Mustard (H, HD, HN), and lewisite (L, HL) are common vesicants. All are very toxic, although much less so than nerve agents. A few drops on the skin can cause severe injury, and three grams absorbed through the skin can be fatal. While some vesicants (such as lewisite) act immediately, clinical symptoms from others may not appear for hours or days. The symptoms of vesicant exposure include:

- Eyes: Reddening, congestion, tearing, burning, and a "gritty" feeling; in severe cases, swelling of the eyelids, severe pain, and spasm of the eyelids.
- Skin: Within one to twelve hours, initial mild itching followed by redness, tenderness, and burning pain, followed by burns and fluid-filled blisters. The effects are enhanced in the warm, moist areas of the groin and armpits.

- Respiratory system: Within two to twelve hours, burning sensation in the nose and throat, hoarseness, profusely running nose, severe cough, and shortness of breath.
- Digestive system: Within two to three hours, abdominal pain, nausea, blood-stained vomiting, and bloody diarrhea.

Vesicant agents are heavy, oily liquids, dispersed by aerosol or vaporization, so small explosions or spray equipment may be present. In a pure state they are nearly colorless and odorless, but slight impurities give them a dark color and an odor suggesting mustard, garlic, or onions. Outward signs of vesicant agents include complaints of eye and respiratory irritation along with reports of a garlic-like odor. Similar symptoms will occur among many individuals exposed.

Cyanogens

Cyanogens interfere with the ability of the blood to transport oxygen and result in asphyxiation. Common cyanogens include hydrogen cyanide (AC) and cyanogen chloride (CK). Cyanide and cyanide compounds are common industrial chemicals with which emergency responders sometimes deal. CK can cause tearing of the eyes and irritate the lungs. All cyanogens are toxic at high concentrations and lead to rapid death. Affected persons require removal to fresh air and respiratory therapy. Clinical symptoms of patients affected by cyanogens include respiratory distress, vomiting and diarrhea, vertigo and headaches.

Under pressure, blood agents are liquids. In pure form, they are gases. Precursor chemicals are typically cyanide salts and acids. All have the aroma of bitter almonds or peach blossoms. They are common industrial chemicals and are readily available.

Pulmonary Agents

Pulmonary agents stress the respiratory tract. Severe distress causes edema (fluid in the lungs), which can result in asphyxiation resembling drowning. Chlorine and phosgene, common industrial chemicals, are choking agents. Clinical symptoms include severe eye irritation and respiratory distress (coughing and choking).

Most people recognize the odor of chlorine. Phosgene has the odor of newly cut hay. As both are gases, they must be stored and transported in bottles or cylinders.

Riot Control Agents

Riot control agents include irritating agents and psychedelic agents. Each of these agents is designed to incapacitate. Generally, they are nonlethal; however, irritating agents can result in asphyxiation under certain circumstances, and psychedelic agents could cause behaviors that lead to death.

Common irritating agents include chloropicrin (PS), mace (CN), tear gas (CS), capsicum/pepper spray, adamsite (DM) and dibenzoxazepine (CR). Clinical symptoms include:

- eyes and throat: burning or irritation and tearing of the eyes
- respiratory system: respiratory distress, coughing, choking, and difficulty breathing
- digestive system: with high concentrations, nausea and vomiting

These agents can cause sometimes severe pain on the skin, especially in moist areas. Most exposed persons report the odor of pepper or tear gas. Outward warning signs include the odor of these agents and the presence of dispensing devices. Many are available over the counter.

Psychedelic agents include lysergic acid diethylamide (LSD), 3-quinuclidinyl benzilate (BZ), and benactyzine. These agents alter the nervous system, thereby causing visual and aural hallucinations, a sense of unreality, and changes in thought processes and behavior. Psychedelic agents (sometimes called psychochemicals) are generally characterized by a slightly delayed onset of symptoms and by persistence of symptoms for a period greatly exceeding exposure time. These agents have the ability to incapacitate victims for a relatively short period with essentially no fatalities. The effects of these agents can be unpredictable, ranging from overwhelming fear and panic to extreme belligerence.

EXPLOSIVE INCIDENTS

The U.S. Department of Transportation defines an explosive as a substance fitting into one of these two categories: (1) Any substance or article, including a device, designed to function by explosion (e.g., an extremely rapid release of gas and heat); or (2) any substance or article, including a device, which, by chemical reaction within itself, can function in a similar manner even if not designed to function by explosion, unless the substance or article is otherwise classified.

It is estimated that 70 percent of all terrorist attacks worldwide involve explosives. It is apparent that bombs are the current weapon of choice among terrorist groups. In addition, thousands of bomb hoaxes are reported each year. Improvised explosive and incendiary devices are designed and assembled to explode and cause fires.

INFORMATION ON SPECIFIC AGENTS

The blast effects of a serious explosion can cause injuries to the lungs, abdomen, and ears. The secondary effects of flying debris, shrapnel, and other projectiles can cause penetrating or blunt trauma and/or burns. A lung injury may present as difficulty breathing and possibly blood-tinged sputum. Abdomen injuries due to blasts usually result in pain, nausea, and vomiting. Ear injuries include a ruptured or irritated eardrum, resulting in temporary or permanent hearing loss; occasionally, loss of balance will also occur from injury to the inner ear.

The following pages contain quick reference guides for biological and chemical agents, followed by more detailed information about many of these agents. The guides were derived from similar guides in the course materials for the *Emergency Response to Terrorism* curriculum of the U.S. Fire Administration, National Fire Academy. Information on explosive or incendiary agents is not included in the guides or detailed information, as the effects of these types of agents are typically the same as with more common incidents involving explosions or fires.

The information contained in these guides and the following pages will be helpful when completing the scenarios in this workbook.

Biological Agent Quick Reference Guide

Disease (Class)	Route of Infection	Incubation Period/ Onset Time	Human-to-Human Transmission	Signs and Symptoms	Decontamination or Infection Control Procedures	Prehospital Care
VIRUSES						
Smallpox (virus)	R, S, DC	10 to 12 days	High	Malaise, fever, rigors, vomiting, headache, backache; 2 to 3 days later, lesions develop into pustular vesicles, more abundant on face and extremities, developing synchronously.	Strict quarantine with respiratory isolation for a minimum of 16 to 17 days following exposure for all contacts. Patients are infectious until all scabs heal.	Supportive care.

V = vector, R = respiratory, D = digestive, DC = direct human-to-human contact, S = skin

Disease (Class)	Route of Infection	Incubation Period/ Onset Time	Human-to-Human Transmission	Signs and Symptoms	Decontamination or Infection Control Procedures	Prehospital Care
Venezuelan equine encephalitis (virus)	R, V	2 to 6 days	Low	Sudden onset, with malaise, spiking fever, rigors, severe headache, photophobia, and myalgia. Nausea, vomiting, cough, sore throat, and diarrhea may follow	Body substance isolation; infectious through mosquito bites.	Analgesics for headache and myalgia; anticonvulsants and respiratory support.

V = vector, R = respiratory, D = digestive, DC = direct human-to-human contact, S = skin

Disease (Class)	Route of Infection	Incubation Period/ Onset Time	Human-to-Human Transmission	Signs and Symptoms	Decontamination or Infection Control Procedures	Prehospital Care
Viral hemorrhagic fevers (virus)	DC, V, ?R	3 to 21 days	Moderate	Fever, easy bleeding, petechiae, hypotension, shock, edema, malaise, myalgia, headache, vomiting, and diarrhea.	Decontamination with hypochlorite or phenolic disinfectants. Body substance isolation required.	Supportive care directed at respiratory and circulatory support.

V = vector, R = respiratory, D = digestive, DC = direct human-to-human contact, S = skin

Disease (Class)	Route of Infection	Incubation Period/ Onset Time	Human-to-Human Transmission	Signs and Symptoms	Decontamination or Infection Control Procedures	Prehospital Care
TOXINS						
Botulinum toxin (toxin)	D, R	24 hours to several days	No	Ptosis, weakness, dizziness, dry mouth and throat, blurred vision and diplopia, dysarthria, dysphonia, and dysphagia, followed by symmetrical descending paralysis and respiratory failure.	0.5% hypochlorite solution and/or soap and water.	Aggressive respiratory support; supportive care for other symptoms.

V = vector, R = respiratory, D = digestive, DC = direct human-to-human contact, S = skin

Disease (Class)	Route of Infection	Incubation Period/ Onset Time	Human-to-Human Transmission	Signs and Symptoms	Decontamination or Infection Control Procedures	Prehospital Care
Staphylococcal enterotoxin B (SEB) (toxin)	D, R	4 to 6 hours	No	Sudden onset, with fever, chills, headache, myalgia, and nonproductive cough. Some may develop respiratory distress and retrosternal pain. If ingested, nausea, vomiting, and diarrhea may result.	0.5% hypochlorite solution and/or soap and water.	Supportive care directed at respiratory support.

V = vector, R = respiratory, D = digestive, DC = direct human-to-human contact, S = skin

Disease (Class)	Route of Infection	Incubation Period/ Onset Time	Human-to-Human Transmission	Signs and Symptoms	Decontamination or Infection Control Procedures	Prehospital Care
Ricin (toxin)	D, R	24 to 72 hours	No	Weakness, fever, cough, and pulmonary edema 8 to 24 hours post-exposure, followed by severe respiratory distress and death from hypoxemia in 36 to 72 hours.	0.5% hypochlorite solution and/or soap and water.	Supportive care with aggressive airway management. Volume replacement of GI fluid loss.

V = vector, R = respiratory, D = digestive, DC = direct human-to-human contact, S = skin

Disease (Class)	Route of Infection	Incubation Period/ Onset Time	Human-to-Human Transmission	Signs and Symptoms	Decontamination or Infection Control Procedures	Prehospital Care
Tricho-thecene mycotoxins (T2) (toxin)	R, S, DC, D	Minutes to hours	No	Skin pain, pruritus, redness, vesicles, necrosis; nose and throat pain, nasal discharge, itching and sneezing, cough, dyspnea, wheezing, chest pain, and hemop-tysis; ataxia, shock, and death.	Soap and water, after clothing has been removed. Eye exposure—copious saline irrigation.	Supportive care directed at respira-tory and circulatory support.

V = vector, R = respiratory, D = digestive, DC = direct human-to-human contact, S = skin

Disease (Class)	Route of Infection	Incubation Period/ Onset Time	Human-to-Human Transmission	Signs and Symptoms	Decontamination or Infection Control Procedures	Prehospital Care
BACTERIA						
Anthrax (bacterium)	S, D, R	1 to 6 days	No, except for cutaneous type	Fever, malaise, fatigue, cough, and mild chest discomfort, followed by severe respiratory distress with dyspnea, diaphoresis, stridor, and cyanosis; shock and death within 24 to 36 hours of severe symptoms.	Body substance isolation precautions, decontamination with low-pressure soap and water wash, then 0.5% hypochlorite solution, then second soap and water wash.	Supportive care according to local protocol.

V = vector, R = respiratory, D = digestive, DC = direct human-to-human contact, S = skin

Disease (Class)	Route of Infection	Incubation Period/ Onset Time	Human-to-Human Transmission	Signs and Symptoms	Decontamination or Infection Control Procedures	Prehospital Care
Cholera (bacterium)	D, DC	1 to 5 days	Rare	Asymptomatic to severe with sudden onset, vomiting, abdominal distension, and pain with little or no fever, followed rapidly by diarrhea. Fluid loss can exceed 5 to 10 liters per day.	Enteric precautions, soap and water washes, and a hypochlorite solution for equipment. Personal contact rarely causes infection.	Supportive care directed at rapid fluid replacement.

V = vector, R = respiratory, D = digestive, DC = direct human-to-human contact, S = skin

Disease (Class)	Route of Infection	Incubation Period/ Onset Time	Human-to-Human Transmission	Signs and Symptoms	Decontamination or Infection Control Procedures	Prehospital Care
Pneumonic plague (bacterium)	V, R	2 to 3 days	High	High fever, chills, headache, hemoptysis, and toxemia, with rapid progression to dyspnea, stridor, and cyanosis; death is due to respiratory failure and circulatory collapse.	Strict isolation precautions. Use of soap and water for personnel decon; heat, UV rays, and disinfectants for equipment.	Supportive care and respiratory and circulatory support.

V = vector, R = respiratory, D = digestive, DC = direct human-to-human contact, S = skin

Disease (Class)	Route of Infection	Incubation Period/ Onset Time	Human-to-Human Transmission	Signs and Symptoms	Decontamination or Infection Control Procedures	Prehospital Care
Bubonic plague (bacterium)	V, R	2 to 10 days	High	High fever, chills, malaise, tender lymph nodes (buboes) may progress to septicemic form, with spread to the CNS, lungs, and elsewhere.	Isolation precautions, secretion and lesion precautions. Use of soap and water for personnel decon; heat, UV rays, or disinfectants for equipment.	Supportive care and respiratory and circulatory support.

V = vector, R = respiratory, D = digestive, DC = direct human-to-human contact, S = skin

Disease (Class)	Route of Infection	Incubation Period/ Onset Time	Human-to-Human Transmission	Signs and Symptoms	Decontamination or Infection Control Procedures	Prehospital Care
Tularemia (bacterium)	V, R, D	2 to 10 days	No	Ulcero-glandular—local ulcer and regional lymphadenopathy, fever, chills, headache, and malaise. Typhoidal or septicemic—fever, headache, malaise, substernal discomfort, weight loss, nonproductive cough.	Secretion and lesion precautions, strict isolation not required. Use of heat or disinfectants renders organism harmless.	Supportive care.

V = vector, R = respiratory, D = digestive, DC = direct human-to-human contact, S = skin

Disease (Class)	Route of Infection	Incubation Period/ Onset Time	Human-to-Human Transmission	Signs and Symptoms	Decontamination or Infection Control Procedures	Prehospital Care
Q-Fever (bacterium)	V, R	2 to 10 days	Rare	Fever, cough, and pleuritic chest pain.	Use of soap and water or a weak 0.5% hypochlorite solution.	Supportive care.

V = vector, R = respiratory, D = digestive, DC = direct human-to-human contact, S = skin

Chemical Agents Quick Reference Guide

Agent Type Civilian (Military) Name	Route of Exposure	Onset of Symptoms	Signs and Symptoms	Decontamination	Prehospital Care
NERVE Tabun (GA) Sarin (GB) Soman (GD) VX	R, S	seconds to 18 hours	Miosis, difficulty breathing, headache, muscular twitching; salivation, lacrimation, urination, defecation, gastrointestinal distress, emesis (SLUDGE); seizures, coma, death	Body substance isolation precautions for responders, decontamination with 0.5% hypochlorite solution, then soap and water wash.	Respiratory support, atropine 2 mg IM, repeat until atropinization occurs; pralidoxime chloride (2-PAM CI) 600 mg, IM maximum prehospital dose 1800 mg; diazepam 10 mg IM repeated according to local protocol.

S = skin absorption, I = ingestion, R = respiratory

Agent Type Civilian (Military) Name	Route of Exposure	Onset of Symptoms	Signs and Symptoms	Decontamination	Prehospital Care
VESICANTS (BLISTER) Nitrogen mustard (H)(HD) (HN1) (HN2)(HN3) Lewisite (L) (HL) Phosgene oxime (CX)	R, S	2 to 24 hours	Tearing or burning eyes, runny nose, sneezing, cough, nosebleed, redness on skin followed by blisters. *Symptoms are delayed but tissue damage occurs within minutes of contamination.*	Body substance isolation precautions for responders, decontamination with 0.5% hypochlorite solution, then soap and water wash.	Aggressive burn management, airway support, and for lewisite, British anti-lewisite. The blister fluid will not contain vesicant agent.

S = skin absorption, I = ingestion, R = respiratory

Agent Type Civilian (Military) Name	Route of Exposure	Onset of Symptoms	Signs and Symptoms	Decontamination	Prehospital Care
CYANOGENS Hydrogen cyanide (AC) Cyanogen chloride (CK)	R, I	15 seconds to 2 minutes	Increased respirations, loss of consciousness seizures, death, *all rapid onset*.	Body substance isolation precautions for responders, decontamination with soap and water wash.	Supportive care and respiratory and circulatory support, use of cyanide antidote kit or IV sodium nitrate and sodium thiosulfate.
PULMONARY (CHOKING)					
Phosgene (CG) Chlorine	R	20 minutes to 24 hours	Eye and airway irritation, dyspnea, chest tightness, bronchospasm, delayed noncardiogenic pulmonary edema.	Body substance isolation precautions for responders, decontamination with soap and water wash.	Supportive care and respiratory and circulatory support. Aggressive airway management, use of intubation with PEEP. ACLS pulmonary edema medications may be ineffective.

S = skin absorption, I = ingestion, R = respiratory

Agent Type Civilian (Military) Name	Route of Exposure	Onset of Symptoms	Signs and Symptoms	Decontamination	Prehospital Care
RIOT CONTROL (IRRITATING) Mace (CN) Tear gas (CS) Pepper spray Adamsite (DM) Dibenzoxazepine (CR)	R, S, I	seconds	Burning pain on mucous membranes, skin, and eyes; tearing, burning in nostrils, elevated blood pressure, irregular respiration, nausea/vomiting from high concentrations. Has been fatal in confined spaces. Symptoms will usually resolve in 15 to 20 minutes after removal to fresh air.	Eyes—flush with water or saline; skin—copious amounts of water, alkaline soap, or mild alkaline solution, sodium bicarbonate or sodium carbonate. *Do not use hypochlorite, which will worsen skin symptoms.*	Supportive care, as the effects are usually self-limiting. May trigger asthma attacks in sensitive patients in a confined space.

S = skin absorption, I = ingestion, R = respiratory

Agent Type Civilian (Military) Name	Route of Exposure	Onset of Symptoms	Signs and Symptoms	Decontamination	Prehospital Care
RIOT CONTROL (PSYCHEDELIC) Lysergic acid diethylamide (LSD) 3-quinuclidinyl benzilate (BZ) Benactyzine	R, I	30 minutes to 24 hours	Visual and aural hallucinations, sense of unreality, changes in thought processes, changes in behavior, ranging from overwhelming fear and panic to extreme belligerence.	Not contagious or infectious from human to human.	Supportive care, as with an overdose patient. Patient may exhibit extreme behavior shifts, so extreme vigilance during treatment and transport is important.

S = skin absorption, I = ingestion, R = respiratory

BIOLOGICAL AGENTS

Smallpox (Virus)

Systemic	Malaise, fever, rigors, vomiting, and backache.
Neurological	Headache.
Pulmonary	No significant effects.
Cutaneous	Within two to three days after onset of prodromal illness, lesions appear that quickly progress from macules to papules and eventually to pustular vesicles. They are more abundant on the extremities and face, and develop synchronously. From eight to fourteen days after onset, the pustules form scabs, which leave depressed depigmented scars upon healing.
Circulatory	No significant effects.
Epidemiology	Incubation period of ten to twelve days.

Venezuelan Equine Encephalitis (Virus)

Systemic	Malaise, spiking fevers, rigors, photophobia, myalgia, nausea, vomiting, sore throat, diarrhea.
Neurological	Severe headache.
Pulmonary	No significant effects.
Cutaneous	No significant effects.
Circulatory	No significant effects.
Epidemiology	No casualties, aerosol dissemination, acute onset.

Viral Hemorrhagic Fevers (Virus)

Systemic	Symptoms can include high fever, headache, myalgias, stomach pain, fatigue, diarrhea, hypotension, and, in the most severe cases, shock and hemorrhage. In some patients, sore throat, hiccups, rash,

	red and itchy eyes, vomiting blood, and bloody diarrhea may also be present.
Neurological	Signs and symptoms can include headache, photophobia, hyperesthesia, confusion, tremor, and visual and auditory hallucinations.
Pulmonary	The onset of illness is abrupt, and initial symptoms resemble those of an influenza-like syndrome, including cough and chest pain in some cases.
Cutaneous	Signs of VHF include conjunctivitis, prominent maculo-papular rashes (particularly for Marburg and Ebola virus diseases) and flushing of the face and chest.
Circulatory	After the third day of illness, hemorrhagic manifestations are common and include petechiae as well as frank bleeding, which can arise from any part of the gastrointestinal tract, mucus membranes, and other multiple sites.

Botulinum Toxin (Toxin)

Systemic	Generalized weakness, dizziness, decreased mobility. Initially, postural hypotension (low blood pressure) may be present.
Neurological	Early ocular symptoms are blurred vision due to mydriasis (dilation of pupil), diplopia (single object perceived as two), ptosis (drooping eyelids), and photophobia (dread and avoidance of light). Other bulbar signs include dysarthria (speech disturbance), dysphonia (altered voice production), and dysphagia (difficulty swallowing). Skeletal muscle flaccid paralysis with symmetrical, descending, progressive weakness follows these bulbar signs. The degree of paralysis varies

	depending on the degree of progression in the patient. Narcosis (stupor) may occur with respiratory muscle paralysis.
Pulmonary	Progressive development of respiratory failure. Early upper respiratory symptoms include dry mouth, sore throat, and absent gag reflex. After development of skeletal muscle paralysis, respiratory failure may abruptly follow.
Cutaneous	Cyanosis may occur with respiratory muscle paralysis.
Circulatory	No significant direct effect.

Staphylococcal Enterotoxin B (Toxin)

Systemic	Fever (103° to 106°F), chills, headache, myalgia (pain in muscles), postural hypotension (fall in blood pressure).
Neurological	No significant effects.
Pulmonary	Pulmonary edema, nonproductive cough, shortness of breath, retrosternal chest pain.
Cutaneous	No significant effects.
Circulatory	No significant effects.
Epidemiology	Symptoms can occur three to twelve hours after aerosol exposure (typically four to six hours). Higher exposure can lead to septic shock and death. Incapacitates 50 percent of those exposed.

Ricin (Toxin)

Systemic	Weakness, fever, nausea, arthralgia (joint pain) eight to twenty-four hours after inhalation exposure.
Neurological	No significant effects.
Pulmonary	Cough, pulmonary edema, severe respiratory distress, chest tightness, dyspnea (labored breathing).
Cutaneous	Cyanosis (blueness of skin).

Circulatory	No significant effects.
Epidemiology	Severe exposure can result in death within thirty-six to seventy-two hours. Anticipate a large number of victims, especially if toxin is aerosolized.

Anthrax (Bacterium)

Systemic	Fever, malaise, and fatigue may be present, sometimes in association with a nonproductive cough and mild chest discomfort. These initial symptoms are often followed by a short period of improvement (hours to two to three days), followed by the abrupt development of severe respiratory distress with dyspnea, diaphoresis, stridor, and cyanosis. Shock and death usually follow within twenty-four to thirty-six hours after the onset of respiratory distress.
Neurological	Meningitis may occur following bacteremia as a complication of any of the clinical forms of the disease. Meningitis may also occur very early, without a clinically apparent primary focus. It is often hemorrhagic, which is almost always fatal.
Pulmonary	Mild, then abruptly severe respiratory signs; possible change in chest appearance, chest congestion, and mild cyanosis of lips. Respiratory signs begin with a nonproductive cough and mild chest discomfort. Chest X-rays may reveal a widened mediastinum with pleural effusions but typically without infiltrates. After the short period of improvement, severe respiratory distress develops abruptly with dyspnea (shortness of breath), diaphoresis, and stridor (high-pitched, noisy respiration). Note: Pulmonary and cutaneous effects do not normally appear together.

Cutaneous	Cyanosis (dark bluish coloration of the skin and mucous membrane) appears with onset of severe symptoms. Cutaneous anthrax (also referred to as malignant pustule) occurs most frequently on the hands and forearms of persons working with infected livestock. It is characterized by an initial papule followed by formation of a blister-like, fluid-filled vesicle. This vesicle typically drops and forms a coal-black scab called an eschar. Sometimes this local infection will develop into a systemic infection, which is often fatal if untreated. Note: Cutaneous and pulmonary effects do not normally appear together.
Circulatory	No significant effects.

Tularemia (Bacterium)

Systemic	Fever, chills, headache and malaise, substernal discomfort, prostration, weight loss.
Neurological	Headache.
Pulmonary	Significant nonproductive cough, pneumonia, substernal chest discomfort.
Cutaneous	Necrotic tender ulcer usually located at site of inoculation; tender, enlarged regional lymph nodes.
Circulatory	No known effects.
Epidemiology	Incubation two to ten days (three to five days most common).

CHEMICAL AGENTS

Tabun (GA) (Nerve)

Systemic	Nausea, vomiting, defecation, and urination.

Neurological	Runny nose, constriction of the pupils (miosis), drooling, twitching and jerking, coma.
Pulmonary	Tightness in the chest, difficulty breathing, suffocation as a consequence of convulsive spasms.
Cutaneous	No cutaneous effects.
Circulatory	No circulatory effects.
Epidemiology	Amber, nonpersistent liquid that gives off little odor when vaporizing. The vapor is colorless. If a person does not receive an immediate lethal dose, death will occur after approximately twenty minutes. People who do not accumulate a lethal dose but do not receive immediate appropriate medical treatment may still suffer permanent neurological damage.

Sarin (GB) and Cyclosarin (Nerve)

Systemic	Vapor, large exposure—copious secretions. Liquid on skin, small to moderate exposure—localized sweating, nausea, vomiting, feeling of weakness. Liquid on skin, large exposure—copious secretions, drooling, stomach cramps, nausea, vomiting, sweating, leading to loss of muscle control, twitching, rhinorrhea, paralysis, unconsciousness, convulsions, coma, and death.
Neurological	Tearing of the eyes within minutes of exposure, eye pain, headache, forgetfulness, difficulty concentrating, irritability, depression, unconsciousness, coma, and death. Dimmed or impaired vision. Vapor, small exposure—miosis (constricted pupils). Vapor, large exposure—sudden loss of consciousness, convulsions, apnea (suspension of breathing), flaccid paralysis,

	miosis. Liquid on skin, large exposure—sudden loss of consciousness, convulsions, apnea (suspension of breathing), flaccid paralysis.
Pulmonary	Vapor, small exposure—mild difficulty breathing, chest tightness.
Cutaneous	No significant effects.
Circulatory	Changes in heart rate.
Epidemiology	Delivery by rocket, mine, or bomb. Sudden onset of symptoms: odorless, colorless.

Soman (GD) (Nerve)

Systemic	Runny nose, nausea, vomiting, uncontrolled defecation and urination.
Neurological	Constriction of the pupils (miosis), drooling, twitching and jerking, coma.
Pulmonary	Tightness in the chest, difficulty breathing, suffocation as a consequence of convulsive spasms.
Cutaneous	No cutaneous effects.
Circulatory	No circulatory effects.
Epidemiology	Colorless liquid, which gives off an odor of rotting fruit when vaporizing. The vapor is colorless. A persistent agent that can easily remain in a particular area for a day or longer, depending on the atmospheric conditions. The thickened soman is a yellowish-brown, highly viscous liquid.

VX (Nerve)

Systemic	Gastrointestinal effects. After absorption, agent causes increase in motility of GI tract and increase in secretions by the glands in the wall of the GI tract. Small amounts will initially cause nausea, vomiting, rhinorrhea, and salivation. Large amounts may cause diarrhea.

Neurological	Skeletal muscle and central nervous system effects. Initial effects of the skeletal muscle may produce muscular fasciculations (involuntary contractions that are visible under the skin) or twitching at the site of the liquid droplet. Large amounts of this agent cause fatigue, weakness, and muscular flaccidity shortly after exposure, and usually cause generalized fasciculations. There may be an asymptomatic period of one to thirty minutes after exposure to a large amount of the agent before it affects the central nervous system. Then loss of consciousness, seizure activity, and apnea (cessation of breathing) occur. Exposure to a small amount may cause forgetfulness, insomnia, irritability, impaired judgment, and/or depression. Additional symptoms are nightmares and difficulty with expression. Exposure to a large amount or exposure close to or in the eye causes severe miosis, pinpointed pupils, and red eyes with tearing.
Pulmonary	Bronchoconstriction, secretions, cough, chest tightness, shortness of breath, wheezing, rales, and rhonchi. VX nerve gas disrupts the functioning of nerves that control breathing. The victim dies of suffocation when the diaphragm fails to expand and contract.
Cutaneous	Localized sweating and blanching. Unlike any other biological or chemical weapons, VX can kill simply by touching the skin and is primarily toxic by the dermal route.
Circulatory	Decrease or increase in heart rate, usually increase in blood pressure.
Epidemiology	Symptoms can occur in a matter of seconds or up to eighteen hours later.

Lewisite (L) (Vesicant)

Systemic	Inhaling the vapors causes painful, long-lasting blisters to form all over the body and results in itchy skin, watery eyes, and burning sensation in lungs. It can also cause blindness. The first symptoms of all blistering agents are reddening of the skin, especially around the eyes, and large water blisters on all exposed areas of skin. Extreme irritation of the respiratory tract may occur if any vapor has been inhaled; eyes may also be damaged. The blisters are very slow to heal and all the time they are vulnerable to infection. Any damage to the respiratory tract can result in chronic long-term respiratory disorders. HL will cause the lung tissues to swell and produce low blood pressure, severe bowel troubles, and a general feeling of weakness and restlessness. The immediate effects of exposure are eye irritation, possibly culminating in permanent eye damage, and reddening of the skin, blisters form after about thirty minutes. A high concentration can cause death within ten minutes.
Neurological	The mustard component of HL causes limited neurological effects similar to nerve agents affecting the acetylcholinesterase. The effects are normally not significant because the concentrations necessary to produce neurological effects would completely overwhelm the victim.
Pulmonary	HL causes pulmonary edema damaging the lung tissue and producing the fluids normally associated with edema.
Cutaneous	Exposure to HL causes immediate erythema (reddening of the skin) with pruritus,

	vomiting or stinging. Within hours, extreme blistering will occur in all exposed areas that were not decontaminated especially in warm, moist areas with thin skin such as perineum, genitalia, axillae, antecubital fossal, and neck.
Circulatory	Damaged blood cells may occur but overall circulatory effects are limited.
Epidemiology	Tissue damage can occur within minutes.

Cyanide (AC) (Cyanogen)

Systemic	The systemic effects associated with AC are generalized malaise, fatigue, and weakness. These symptoms appear only with extremely low exposure. At high exposure, the principal effects will cause death without the manifestation of systemic effects.
Neurological	Headache, vertigo, anxiousness, sluggish pupils. General CNS excitement including anxiety, personality changes, agitation, and seizures. Unresponsive coma and dilated pupils.
Pulmonary	Transient, rapid breathing. Gasping, inability to hold breath. Inability of red blood cells to process oxygen.
Cutaneous	Diaphoresis, flushing, normally cherry red skin.
Circulatory	Vascular flush.
Epidemiology	Onset of symptoms can occur in fifteen seconds to two minutes.

Phosgene (CG) (Pulmonary)

Systemic	CG's systemic effects include malaise and fatigue as with other agents. However, the concentrations associated with field exposure make the systemic effects limited.

Neurological	No neurological effects.
Pulmonary	Phosgene attacks the respiratory tract (nose, throat, and lungs), causing membranes to swell and filling the lungs with fluids so the victim drowns. Victims who survive an exposure are likely to suffer chronic breathing troubles for the rest of their lives. For low exposure—mild cough, chest discomfort, and dyspnea. For high exposure—pulmonary edema, severe cough, dyspnea, frothy sputum, laryngospasm, and sudden cough.
Cutaneous	Phosgene CG does not harm the skin.
Circulatory	No circulatory effects.
Epidemiology	Onset of symptoms in twenty minutes to twenty-four hours, depending upon exposure and individual level of fitness/wellness.

Chlorine (Pulmonary)

Systemic	Rhinorrhea, epistaxis, choking or cough, swallowing difficulties, stridor, hoarseness, aphonia. Retching and vomiting.
Neurological	Burning, itching, tearing, painful eyes. Diffuse or focal neurological dysfunction.
Pulmonary	Damage to respiratory tract, cellular damage with consequent airway obstruction, pulmonary interstitial damage. Nasal irritation. Wheezing, substernal burning, dyspnea, chest tightness. Suffocation (inability to get enough air). Rapidly increasing choking sensation. Dyspnea (shortness of breath).
Cutaneous	Cyanosis.
Circulatory	Palpitations, angina, syncope.
Epidemiology	Aerosol, particles, either liquid or solid suspended in air. Mist, fumes, smokes and

dust. Distinct odor. Greenish-yellow gas. Settles in low-lying areas.

Lysergic Acid Diethylamide (LSD), Benactyzine, and 3-Quinuclidinyl Benzilate (BZ) (Psychedelic)

Systemic	Thirst, decreased bladder tone and decreased urinary force, severe bladder distention, muscle weakness, heightened stretch reflexes.
Neurological	Stupor, confusion, confabulation with concrete and panoramic illusions and hallucinations, and with regression to automatic "phantom" behaviors such as plucking and disrobing. Mydriasis (blurred vision), dry mouth, disorientation regarding time and place. Disturbances in judgment and insight. Patient may revert to vulgar and inappropriate behavior. Patient may be readily distracted and may have memory loss and posthallucinogenic amnesia. Patient has slurred and senseless speech and appears intoxicated.
Pulmonary	No pulmonary effects.
Cutaneous	Decreased stimulation of eccrine and apocrine sweat glands in the skin result in dry, beet-red skin. Skin becomes warm to hot.
Circulatory	Initially rapid heart rate; later, normal or slow heart rate.
Epidemiology	Psychochemical agent typically distributed by an aerosol. Agent is odorless and nonirritating; effects are not seen for thirty minutes to twenty-four hours. The agent is persistent. Hallucinogenic effects are more pronounced than its potent hypotensive properties.

RADIOLOGICAL AGENTS

Radiological/Nuclear

Systemic	Gastrointestinal effects from low exposure are nausea and vomiting. High exposure causes GI ulceration and bleeding, diarrhea, and intestinal disorders. Other signs are lethargy, hair loss, sterilization, nosebleed, and fever.
Neurological	Effects on the central nervous system from high exposure occur within one to forty-eight hours. They include seizures, loss of muscle coordination (twitching, cramps/spasms, and convulsions), coma, lethargy, and tremors.
Pulmonary	Although the pulmonary system is not significantly affected by radiation directly, the body has an overall decreasing ability to fight off disease due to the jeopardization of the immuno-response system. Other pulmonary symptoms include rhinorrhea, wheezing, cough, and sore throat.
Cutaneous	A transient prodromal erythema occurs within minutes to hours after exposure and may disappear within thirty-six hours. During the manifestational state, which occurs with a latency period of seven to twenty-one days, the symptoms range from bright erythemas with a sensation of burning to blisters and ulcers, which may be extremely painful. After high doses of radiation, there may even be a total epidermal necrolysis resembling Lyell's syndrome. In the subacute stage, initiation of dermal and subcutaneous fibrosis leads to a second ulcerative phase and cutaneous ischemia in the affected areas.
Circulatory	Hematopoietic effects from low exposure occur in four to six weeks and include a

	decrease in white blood cells, hemorrhage, infection, elevated pulse, decreased blood pressure, and electrolyte imbalance.
General Effects	Loss of blood-forming organs, infection, anemia, loss of cells lining the intestines, diarrhea, electrolyte imbalance, loss of muscle coordination, seizures, coma, skin burns.
Epidemiology	The onset of symptoms varies depending on the type and amount of radiation to which a victim is exposed. Low exposure is one to three hours; high exposure is five to fourteen days. Nuclear flesh burns are normally immediate. Radiation effects appear within hours after exposure. For a radiological device, the victim had to be physically present in the contaminated area.

4 Terrorism Emergency Response Scenarios

INSTRUCTIONS

The basic instructions for completing these scenarios are to identify at a minimum the agent category and, if possible, the specific agent that was most likely used in the incident. In some cases, it will be impossible to narrow the type to a single agent; however, the same is true in real-world situations. In other scenarios, no agent was used.

These scenarios can be used for different purposes and by different types of responders—fire, rescue, EMS, haz-mat, and law enforcement personnel. The scenarios can also be used with a variety of methodologies or with expanded instructions. For example, an individual working to increase his/her understanding of the effects of terrorist incidents may use these to study the effects of individual biological and chemical agents. On the other hand, an instructor can use these scenarios for class discussion questions, for homework, or as test questions related to product identification, treatment modalities, development of strategy and tactics, or incident action planning. To help organize the diverse ways these scenarios can be administered, a matrix indicating which scenarios fall into the agent categories of biological, chemical, radiological, or explosive agents can be found in Appendix A.

In addition to category or product identification, other activities to consider for each scenario are:

- Identify the outward warning signs.
- Identify the primary type of harm that can be expected to have already occurred at the incident.
- Identify and describe the secondary types of harm that may be present.
- Identify methods of self-protection that could be used.

- List method(s) for detecting and monitoring the material suspected.
- Identify and describe tactical considerations that may be implemented.
- List the technical resources available at the local, state, and federal levels.
- Develop an Incident Command System chart for the overall response to the given scenario.

Because of the varying factors involved with any type of scenario (audience, resource availability, environmental and weather, conditions, population density, etc.), expanded answers among those completing the scenarios could vary significantly, depending upon where the individual lives, their level of training and expertise, and their background. For example, a twenty-year veteran battalion chief in a major metropolitan fire department may have different considerations in any of the scenarios compared to those of a new EMT in a rural volunteer fire department or a state police trooper. None of their answers may be wrong, but the answers will all come from a different perspective. Because of this, only the identification of the agent category and/or agent(s) most likely involved is provided as a solution to the scenarios. These solutions can be found in Appendix B.

SCENARIOS

1. You are startled by a large explosion that seemed to be only a few blocks away. You respond immediately to investigate and receive a report that a van has exploded. As you arrive, victims are everywhere. Some are choking and wheezing; others are complaining of substernal burning. In addition to injuries from the explosion, you notice that many of the victims have bloody noses, while others can't talk. All victims are rubbing their eyes, complaining that they itch and burn. Those who can talk report an overwhelming choking sensation immediately after the explosion.

2. An explosion occurred about eighteen hours ago. The victims of the explosion report having been sprayed with a smelly liquid from one or possibly two bombs. Their skin began to hurt within a few minutes. Within about six hours, their skin started itching. They also report having a burning sensation in the chest.

3. You are at the fire station in a popular resort town when you learn of an attack on a group of tourists. You arrive on the scene within thirty minutes. Two victims closest to the explosion have already died after first having convulsions. Those who are left have runny noses and are complaining of chest tightness. You also notice a constriction of the pupils of their eyes. Some of the victims have lost control over their bodily functions. Others are twitching and jerking, and four have started convulsing. There was reportedly a very slightly fruity odor after the explosion.

4. You are at the local training center with your engine company when you learn of an explosion in the center of the city. When you arrive at the scene, you notice that there are hundreds of victims, some already dead. Those victims still alive are experiencing severe eye pain as well as nausea and vomiting. Victims who were not close to the explosion are experiencing runny noses and some drooling.

5. You have just arrived for duty at General Hospital when several patients arrive with flulike symptoms. When questioned, one patient reports seeing an unusual cloud over the city the previous day. None of the patients noticed an odor. There are rumors that weapons testing has been conducted in the desert about thirty kilometers from town.

6. Numerous medical facilities within your community are suddenly overtaxed by an inexplicable influx of patients, all presenting with similar symptoms, including weakness, fever, cough, and pulmonary edema. All of these patients visited a local mall during the past forty-eight hours.

7. Five days ago you were dispatched for a warehouse fire on the outskirts of town. Upon arriving you discovered that several large dumpsters were on fire. Neighbors indicated that they heard several explosions before seeing the smoke and calling the fire department. Neighbors of the warehouse are now being brought into the hospital with acute onset of fever, myalgia, malaise, and diffuse bleeding from the gums and eyes. Several of the victims went into shock and died upon arrival at the hospital.

8. You receive a call that a transformer has exploded. Upon arriving at the scene, you find the transformer untouched, but a building housing an abortion clinic has been damaged, with debris scattered over a large area. There is no fire.

9. You have just sat down for lunch at the station when an alarm is dispatched for an explosion at the Bosnian Embassy, where there are several fatalities and multiple injuries. Upon arrival you encounter a large number of victims, most of them lying down vomiting and twitching. Others are complaining of severe stomach pain.

10. You are dispatched to a shooting at a Catholic church across town. When you arrive at the scene, several victims are already dead. Others are drooling and have runny noses. Those close to the attack have watery eyes, impaired vision, and are beginning to twitch and jerk. Those farthest from the attack have headaches. Witnesses report seeing rockets flying into the building.

11. You are at the fire station to start your twenty-four-hour shift when you learn of an incident that occurred last night on 3rd Street downtown. During roll call, you are told that about ten fire and EMS personnel from station 3 were taken to the hospital about twelve hours after the incident. All of the victims have respiratory distress, cough, and fever. Most of the victims are nauseous and have bluish-colored skin. All of the personnel said that they heard a popping sound followed by an aerosol cloud as company 10 arrived on the scene. When asked if there was an odor associated with the cloud, each victim responds "no."

12. You are on duty in the ER when about twenty victims arrive late one night. Most of them are complaining of similar symptoms, including vomiting and diarrhea. One of the men says that there was a loud "bang" about forty-five minutes earlier near their apartment building. When they went to investigate, they noticed a liquid in the area. One victim arrived without symptoms, but while you are examining the other patients she suddenly collapses and starts to convulse.

13. Several victims arrived at the local hospital late last night with reddened skin and complaints of burning in their lungs. By that afternoon, some of the victims also have blisters on their arms. The victims do not want anyone to touch their eyes. Some of them just keep their eyes closed and become very upset when they are examined. During the investigation, they describe sounds of fireworks that were accompanied by a strange odor last night.

14. A call is received from the town's U.S. Post Office reporting an explosion. The first unit arrives at the scene and reports that several postal workers are suffering from minor injuries. The postmaster reports that a loud explosion occurred in the parcel package section, and debris was scattered in all directions. Twenty-three workers and an unknown number of customers were inside the post office at the time of the explosion.

15. The town's emergency communication center received a call from a bailiff at the local courthouse. The bailiff reported that powdery material had been coming out of the vents inside the courthouse building. When he went to investigate, he found two individuals pouring a white powder from a pint jar into the air ducts. He placed the subjects under arrest, and when he questioned them, they stated that everyone in the courthouse was going to die. They wouldn't say what the material was, other than to say that they made the material themselves using beans, and got the recipe off the Internet.

16. On your way to work at General Hospital, you learn from your supervisor that over a thousand people began arriving at area hospitals early this morning. The patients all have fever, malaise, and nonproductive cough. Many patients are experiencing increasing chest discomfort and dyspnea. A few patients have died from shock. The victims all live in the same area of the city and report that they heard low-flying planes three nights ago.

17. You are the health and safety officer of a large combination fire department. About three days ago, you learned that the doctors in the local hospital treated a firefighter for acute onset of high fever, malaise, and cough with bloody sputum. When you spoke to the others in her station, you learned that at least three more firefighters came in with similar symptoms about two days ago and are progressively getting worse. Today, two firefighters died from respiratory failure and circulatory collapse. The firefighters report that they were involved in a house fire five days ago and heard several strange-sounding explosions coming from one corner of the basement as they worked in the basement during overhaul.

18. You are on duty at the hospital when you get a report that there has been an accident at the International Airport. As the victims start to arrive at the hospital, they seem to be exhibiting similar symptoms. Most of the victims are choking and complaining of burning in their chests. Several victims are bleeding profusely from the nose, while others are retching and vomiting. Each victim has burning, itchy, tearing eyes as well. About an hour later, you learn that there was a greenish-yellow gas with a distinct odor that has settled in the low-lying areas near the airport.

19. In a large southern city, there is a van explosion near the waterfront during the noon hour. As you arrive at the scene, you notice that more than fifty victims are already dead. Others are vomiting and drooling. When you examine one of the victims, she is irritable and has difficulty concentrating when you ask her questions about the explosion. You notice that her pupils are constricted just before she goes into convulsions.

20. You are in a large Midwestern city for a meeting when you hear that a terrorist attack on the conference is planned. As you leave for the conference one morning, you hear a loud explosion and see a flash of light in the distance. Expecting mass casualties, you rush to volunteer your service at the closest hospital. Within an hour many patients begin arriving. They are vomiting and have reddened skin.

21. You are dispatched to a riot that occurred during a peace rally. The police department advised that a man wearing a gas mask drove a jeep through the riot and released an aerosolized cloud behind it. Upon arriving at the command post, you are told that approximately ten people were injured. After several hours on the scene monitoring the incident, you find that over half the people involved in the riot are complaining of headaches and sore muscles. Some of the injured appear out of breath with retrosternal chest pain; one dies a short time later.

22. You are on your way to headquarters when you learn of a situation at the city library. Cans of a yellowish-brown liquid have apparently been left in corners of the library. Patrons and others are streaming out of the building. When you arrive about fifteen minutes later, the scene is chaotic. As you begin to examine victims, you notice that several have constricted pupils, rhinorrhea, stomach cramps, and chest tightness.

23. You are on your way to the "East Meets West" conference when you learn about an explosion in the downtown area. Several minutes after the explosion, victims began to arrive at the hospital. When you begin to talk with victims, they tell you that shortly after the explosion, several people went into convulsions and died. Some people smelled a strange odor. The victims who survived are complaining of headaches, vertigo, and malaise; some have flushed skin.

24. You are dispatched for a fire and explosion in an apartment building. Initial reports state that there was an explosion in a fourth floor apartment in a predominantly immigrant area of town. The report also states that the victims began to exhibit similar symptoms immediately, and several are already dead. Before the victims died, they had convulsions. Those victims who were within several blocks of the explosion have runny noses and constricted pupils (miosis). Many of the victims are having breathing difficulties and are drooling. Some casualties reported a perfume-like fragrance; others smelled nothing.

25. You are on duty as the battalion chief in a large city when you get a report of a car bomb on the outskirts of the city. Fortunately, nobody was very close to the car, but three firefighters who responded to put out the fire as well as several police officers who came to investigate are beginning to show unusual symptoms. You are sent to the hospital to interview and check on the fire department personnel. As you arrive at the hospital, you see victims who have runny noses, chest tightness, and constricted pupils (miosis). As you begin to interview the victims, you notice that some of them are having breathing difficulties and nausea and are drooling. No one remembers any unusual odors during or after fire extinguishment.

26. Your EMS unit is on its way to a staging area in support of a building collapse response operation that occurred three days ago near the center of town. Eyewitnesses reported that there was a muted explosion, followed by a large cloud drifting downwind over the business section of the city. After arriving in staging you are sent to the triage area, where you see many victims with difficulty talking, seeing, and swallowing.

27. You are on your way to a training exercise when you get an order to report to the state university on the other side of the state because of an explosion. When you arrive four hours later, you learn that the explosion was followed by a pleasant grassy odor like a field. There was no cloud or liquid associated with the bomb. All of the victims are experiencing shortness of breath as they try to explain what happened. Several others are vomiting. Three victims have gone into shock and one has already died from respiratory failure.

28. You have been dispatched to the Latvian Embassy for several ill subjects. After examining the patients, you find out that a strange explosion occurred several days ago in the embassy building. No one was injured in the explosion, and it was kept low-key. Several other paramedics are examining other ill embassy workers; the common complaint is acute onset of fever, flushed face, and petechial hemorrhages of the oropharynx. You later find out that a terrorist group claims responsibility for the attack.

29. You are the medical director of a statewide haz-mat response team and are requested to go immediately to County Hospital. They have had more than three hundred patients within the last few hours complaining of two to three days of cough, malaise, fever, and chest discomfort. More than seventy-five patients have gone into shock and died. Antibiotics have not been helpful in those severely symptomatic patients. On your way to the hospital, one of the radio stations announces that there were reports of low-flying aircraft over the city five nights ago.

30. Friday evening at 6:00 P.M., your emergency communications center receives a call from a local hospital that it is undertaking emergency evacuation as numerous people are falling ill for no apparent reason. Symptoms include blurred vision, muscular convulsions, and profound tearing and nasal discharge.

31. While investigating an explosion that took place five days earlier at a major sporting event, you learn that twenty-seven civilians who were near the explosion are now complaining of severe headache and muscle aches that began one to three days ago. Most of the victims are blinking and squinting in the light. Several of the patients who have been sick the longest are also beginning to complain of nausea, vomiting, and cough. You find out later that all the victims reported seeing an odorless cloud following the explosion.

32. You are dispatched for a sick person. When you arrive, your patient says that he has just returned from a military conference in Pakistan. He is complaining of the flu and is nauseated and continually vomiting. When talking with you, he suggests that there were rumors of weapons testing during his visit. However, he did not see anything unusual.

33. You have just come on shift as part of the Incident Management Team of a large wildland fire. As you arrive at the Incident Command Post, you learn that thirty-six firefighters and civilians are being treated at the medical unit complaining of fever, malaise, and cough. A few are experiencing chest discomfort and severe respiratory distress, and some are cyanotic. The victims report that a plane was flying very low three days ago upwind of their position north of the fire area; the plane looked different than the air tankers being used at the incident.

34. You respond to the local high school following a report of several sick people. A person identified as the principal tells you that a troubled student has claimed he detonated aerosol bomblets two days ago in the school's ventilation system. Over sixty students are beginning to complain of fever, malaise, and nonproductive cough.

35. You are on duty during a large sporting event when you hear a loud explosion. Several casualties at the scene are wheezing and complaining of shortness of breath. The victims who were close to the blast are having some nausea and diarrhea. Many of the victims appear to be weak.

36. You are on duty in midtown preparing dinner when you are dispatched for a sick person in the subway station. You know the subway station will be crowded, since it is still the evening rush hour. While responding, dispatch notifies you that reports indicate that several "attackers" wearing masks sprayed people exiting subway cars. Additional EMS units and police are dispatched. As the victims emerge from the subway, a few have runny noses and are drooling, and many are vomiting. However, many of the sprayed commuters report feeling "just fine." You notice one victim begin to twitch and jerk. Over the course of the next twenty minutes, three evacuated victims suddenly collapse, stop breathing, and convulse.

37. You are the National Fire Academy taking a two-week class when you get a call to report back to your department immediately. While returning home, you learn that the hospitals in the area have been rapidly filling up with patients for the past two days. The authorities do not know if the symptoms the patients are exhibiting are due to a terrorist attack. All of the patients have nonproductive cough, fever, chills, and sudden weight loss. As you gain more information, you learn that a small airplane was spotted downtown five days ago releasing a cloud or spray of some type.

38. You are dispatched to assist a local city on a mass casualty incident. When you arrive at the scene, you learn of a series of explosions that occurred about forty-five minutes earlier in a heavily populated area of the city. Your patients all appear to have reddened skin and are complaining of thirst. When you try to assess the situation, the victims appear confused and are slurring their speech. Two of the casualties subsequently die.

39. You are on your way with an EMS task force to assist an out-of-state city because of an explosion. Terrorists have claimed responsibility, and law enforcement agencies from all over the state have been deployed. Most victims of the explosion are experiencing a burning sensation in their lungs as well as irritated eyes. When you arrive about eight hours later, some victims have begun to blister. Those farther away from the explosion have reddened skin. As you talk to the victims, you learn that there was an odor associated with the blast. Some thought it smelled like garlic or horseradish.

40. Your city is recovering from a terrorist attack that occurred six days ago. As the days pass, your department receives reports of multiple firefighters and civilians with sudden onset of spiking fevers, headaches, myalgia, and photophobia. When asked what they heard and saw, the victims agree that they heard several strange hissing sounds during the attack. There is a lot of confusion and a couple of civilians have already died. It is reported that many animals and rats within the city limits have been found dead.

41. You arrive for work at the airport fire station shortly before midnight. As you watch a plane land, you hear the sound of dull, muffled explosions near the baggage handling area. You rush to the gate area and arrive within a few minutes. Many people have watery eyes and are coughing in addition to a general feeling of weakness and restlessness. As you report in, you notice a dark, oily liquid on the ground, but don't smell anything except the garlic and spices from the nearby restaurants.

42. An army base is attacked by a truck bomb; you arrive about an hour later. Soldiers have already been streaming into the base hospital with similar symptoms: They feel tired and weak even though they have not been involved in any strenuous exercises. Many report headaches.

43. Several paramedics who were on a structure fire four days earlier have reported to the hospital with the same symptoms: nonproductive cough, depression, and weakness. Many have a fever as well. They state that there were popping sounds accompanied by an aerosol cloud in the area where they were working on several occupants injured during the fire.

44. You have just left your job at the local hospital when you get an emergency call to report back to work immediately. On your way to the hospital you learn of an explosion close to the river. There have been several deaths from the blast along with many other casualties. Those who died first went into convulsions.

45. You are dispatched to the local college following reports of an accident near the dormitory area involving a liquid spilled on the ground. Two people are already dead and others are suffering life-threatening symptoms. As you approach the victims, you notice that all of them are vomiting, drooling, and twitching. As you start to examine them, you notice that their pupils are constricted and they are pressing their hands against their chests, complaining of tightness.

46. The town's emergency communications center received a call from the principal at the local high school reporting a fire in the boys' bathroom on the second floor of the two-story school. All nine hundred students and teachers have been evacuated. The first arriving engine company reports gray smoke coming from a side door. The firefighters enter the building with full protective equipment and SCBA, advancing a hoseline. When the ambulance arrives, EMS personnel are directed to several students who are coughing, vomiting, and squinting. Division 2, on the second floor, reports via radio to the incident commander that there is no evidence of any fire and that they are exiting the building. As they exit, they complain of intense skin irritation. When they remove their SCBA facepieces, they also start complaining of burning eyes.

47. You are on your way to attend a fire expo when you learn of an explosion at the conference center. It is cold and snowing that day and some victims were sprayed with liquid from the explosion. The next day several victims are in shock and one has died of respiratory failure.

48. You are called to the scene of a vehicle crash involving a van. One of the occupants of the van fled on foot after the crash. The second occupant was ejected during the crash and is unconscious next to the vehicle. When you look in the rear of the van, you see a package approximately 12 inches × 12 inches × 8 inches. There are thick rubber gloves and a very thick and heavy apron in the back as well.

49. A large Northwestern city is faced with demonstrations and terrorist activities against the World Trade Organization conference. There has been an explosion close to a major tourist attraction. You arrive at the scene within thirty minutes of the explosion. The victims appear to be disoriented and their speech is slurred. Some are complaining of dry skin and thirst. The victims say there were no unusual odors in the aftermath of the blast.

50. You are on your way to the West Coast for an emergency services conference when you learn of a possible terrorist attack ten hours ago near you destination. As you arrive in the city, you are told that dozens of victims are just beginning to arrive at the local hospital, complaining of severe respiratory distress, cough, nausea, and a fever. You also learn that all of the victims recall a hissing sound followed by formation of an odorless aerosol cloud near the site of the incident.

51. Fire headquarters has received reports of an outbreak of nonspecific flulike symptoms in the city. Additionally, some patients are beginning to develop a papular rash on the face, hands, and forearms. The hospital reports that the patients had a prodrome of fever, rigors, nausea, vomiting, headache, and backache. Two weeks earlier, a riot occurred downtown during a peacekeeping demonstration. Several organizations had threatened to launch "a strike at the heart of America" with a "plague" like the one that originated in Egypt in the twelfth century B.C.

52. A nearby city suffers a possible terrorist attack: a loud explosion followed by a strange aerosol cloud. Almost all of the emergency personnel involved have been affected by the attack. They are complaining of respiratory distress and chest tightness. Most of the personnel are coughing and a few are complaining of nausea. There were no unusual odors during the incident. About thirty-six hours after the explosion, five of the emergency personnel die.

53. You are in a city planning meeting when you learn of an incident involving an explosion. Five days later, you begin to hear that many emergency personnel from your department have been checking into the local hospital. All of the victims complain of difficulty seeing in the sunlight, severe headaches, and spiking fevers. As yet there have been no fatalities. All of the personnel reported hearing a loud explosion followed by an odorless cloud during the incident. They say they began to feel sick one to two days ago.

54. You respond to a report of multiple casualties from an unknown cause near the army base just outside of town. When you arrive, you find the victims are choking, coughing, and rubbing their eyes. Many victims look as if they have been crying. Others are retching and vomiting. Two are already dead. As reports come in, you learn that there was a greenish-yellow gas with a distinct odor that has settled in the low-lying areas near the base.

55. You are at a conference in California when you are approached by one of the doctors about an unusual number of patients who have been coming into the hospitals in San Francisco. They all complain of extreme fatigue and many have sores in their mouths. When you interview them, you learn they were all in the desert about ten days previously near an abandoned military training facility.

56. An incident occurred in the subway in a large eastern city. By the next day, many people have been hospitalized and some are developing a cough with white frothy sputum. Victims reported smelling an unusual odor in the subway. Someone saw a person put down a canister that could have been the source of an exposure.

57. You are on your way to a local military base for a joint haz-mat training exercise when you learn of an "accident": an explosion close to the base. Those close to the explosion died after going into convulsions. The victims you see three hours later have runny noses, chest tightness, and constricted pupils (miosis). Those who were closer to the explosion are having difficulty breathing, sweating profusely, drooling, twitching, and experiencing nausea.

58. There has been a large outbreak of illness among workers in the state capitol building. As you examine the patients, you notice that each has a pustular rash, mostly on the face and extremities. Most patients said they had malaise, fever, rigors, vomiting, headache, and backaches a couple of days before the lesions appeared. An extremist group had reportedly threatened the state government two weeks earlier with "total annihilation" if certain political actions weren't taken.

59. Two weeks ago there was rioting in several areas of the city with multiple fires and casualties. As the riots were ending, a low-flying aircraft dropped multiple bomblets over the entire downtown area. After two weeks of cleaning up and investigating the situation, there has been a large outbreak of chickenpox. Victims have been presenting with pustular lesions most prominent on the face and extremities. They complained of an initial onset of fever, rigors, and headache for about two days prior to the rash.

60. During a disturbance at the airport, aerosol canisters emitted a cloudy spray. After the commotion subsided and the airport cleared out, about six hours after the disturbance, about half of the thirty-five passengers involved were complaining of fever, chills, and headache. Several of the passengers appeared short of breath. About twelve hours after the disturbance, three of the passengers went into septic shock and died. All of the other passengers became ill within twenty-four hours of the disturbance but remained stable.

61. After arriving for your shift, you hear reports of an explosion in a crowded resort area nearby, and about twenty minutes later you are dispatched to assist with patient transport. When you arrive on the scene, you notice that some of the victims have reddened skin and are thirsty. One of the victims is slurring her speech when she tries to tell you that there was an explosion in the lobby of the hotel where she was staying. She says that all she saw was smoke and debris, and noticed no unusual smell.

62. You arrive at the station for your shift. As you enter the building, the captain and several firefighters from the last shift walk into the engine bay gasping for breath. They say that they just had experienced a suffocating odor. Some thought it smelled like newly cut grass. The victims are having trouble catching their breath and some are vomiting.

63. You are called to the grounds of a public festival in response to a reported explosion with multiple casualties. The explosive detonated under a performance stage just prior to a major performance.

64. You are en route to work at a nearby air force base when you hear reports that a flood of soldiers has just arrived at the base hospital, shaken and unable to catch their breath. The first patient you see concurs with reports from others of an artillery bombardment as they were marching on base. He also states that there was a peculiar odor, almost like almonds, following the bombardment. The patient says that he has a headache and has trouble keeping his balance while walking.

65. You are responding to an explosion at the multiplex cinema located near a large shopping mall. The cinema building is detached from the mall but is located in the same parking lot. The dispatch center has advised you of numerous reports of injuries in the lobby and among occupants evacuating the building.

66. You are on duty when you hear a loud explosion that appears to be outside the city, but loud enough to be heard. You see a bright light. Within a few hours, a flood of patients arrives at local hospitals. All of the patients have reddened skin and several have bloody noses. As more victims arrive, there are complaints of gastrointestinal pain. Most victims are vomiting.

67. You are dispatched to the British Embassy for a possible chemical release that began about ten hours earlier. As you arrive at the embassy, you learn that small aerosol bomblets were used in the ventilation system of the building. Over 250 victims appeared at triage and most had fever, chills, headache, and sore muscles. A few were short of breath. About four hours after your arrival, five of the victims go into septic shock and die.

68. About one half hour ago, a vehicle parked at the local mall exploded, killing twelve people. As victims start to pour into the hospital where you are located, they tell you that the explosion dispersed a liquid. All of the victims have runny noses and are drooling. Others have started to vomit. The person you are examining is complaining about tightness in his chest.

69. You are on your way to fire headquarters when you are told that several firefighters have just checked into the city general hospital with simultaneous onset of similar symptoms: They are all experiencing high fevers, cough, and severe prostration. As you investigate the situation, the firefighters tell you that they were out on the wildland fire that occurred four days ago near the Alaskan pipeline, in a remote wooded area. They all recalled a sudden release of an odorless aerosol cloud from a device that was lying on the ground. The firefighters didn't think much of it. Due to the severity of the wildland fire, they continued with suppression efforts.

70. A possible terrorist attack occurred during the morning rush hour yesterday in a downtown subway station. Within eight hours after the attack, hundreds of victims and several fire and EMS personnel began arriving at area hospitals complaining of high fever, nausea, chest tightness, and difficulty breathing. Many of the victims were coughing and had bluish skin. The victims you examined stated that there was a popping sound coming from an abandoned backpack in the subway station followed by a spray device releasing an odorless aerosol cloud in the subway. About thirty-six hours after the attack, you learn that several victims have died.

A

Matrix of Scenario Numbers and Agent Categories

Scenario Number by Agent Type

Biological	Chemical	Radiological	Explosive
6	2	1	5
7	3	19	8
11	4	24	14
15	9	35	20
16	10	44	32
17	12	49	48
21	13		55
26	18		63
28	22		65
29	23		66
31	25		
33	27		
34	30		
37	36		
40	38		
43	39		
50	41		
51	42		
52	45		
53	46		
58	47		
59	54		
60	56		
67	57		
69	61		
70	62		
	64		
	68		

B Solutions to Scenarios

1. Explosive with chemical—chlorine
2. Chemical—lewisite (HL)/mustard
3. Chemical—soman (GD)
4. Chemical—sarin (GB)/cyclosarin
5. Radiological
6. Biological—ricin
7. Biological—viral hemorrhagic fever
8. Explosive
9. Chemical—nerve (VX)
10. Chemical—sarin (GB)/cyclosarin
11. Biological—ricin
12. Chemical—nerve (VX)
13. Chemical—lewisite (HL)/mustard
14. Explosive
15. Biological—ricin
16. Biological—anthrax
17. Biological—anthrax
18. Chemical—chlorine
19. Explosive with chemical—sarin (GB)/cyclosarin
20. Radiological
21. Biological—staphylococcal enterotoxin B
22. Chemical—soman (GD)
23. Chemical—cyanide (AC)
24. Explosive with chemical—tabun (GA) or soman (GD)

25. Chemical—tabun (GA)
26. Biological—botulinum toxin
27. Chemical—phosgene (CG)
28. Biological—viral hemorrhagic fever
29. Biological—anthrax
30. Chemical—sarin (GB)/cyclosarin
31. Biological—Venezuelan equine encephalitis
32. Radiological
33. Biological—anthrax
34. Biological—anthrax
35. Explosive with chemical—nerve (VX)
36. Chemical—sarin (GB)/cyclosarin
37. Biological—tularemia
38. Chemical—lysergic acid diethylamide (LSD), 3-quinuclidinyl benzilate (BZ), or benactyzine
39. Chemical—lewisite (HL)/mustard
40. Biological—Venezuelan equine encephalitis
41. Chemical—lewisite (HL)
42. Chemical—cyanide (AC)
43. Biological—tularemia
44. Explosive with chemical—tabun (GA) or sarin (GB)/cyclosarin
45. Chemical—tabun (GA) or soman (GD)
46. Chemical—irritating
47. Chemical—phosgene (CG)
48. Radiological
49. Explosive with chemical—lysergic acid diethylamide (LSD), 3-quinuclidinyl benzilate (BZ), or benactyzine
50. Biological—ricin
51. Biological—smallpox
52. Biological—ricin

53. Biological—Venezuelan equine encephalitis
54. Chemical—chlorine
55. Radiological
56. Chemical—phosgene (CG)
57. Chemical—soman (GD)
58. Biological—smallpox
59. Biological—smallpox
60. Biological—staphylococcal enterotoxin B
61. Chemical—lysergic acid diethylamide (LSD), 3-quinuclidinyl benzilate (BZ), or benactyzine
62. Chemical—phosgene (CG)
63. Explosive
64. Chemical—cyanide (AC)
65. Explosive
66. Radiological
67. Biological—staphylococcal enterotoxin B
68. Chemical—tabun (GA) or soman (GD)
69. Biological—tularemia
70. Biological—ricin

C Bibliography

Almond, George. "The Manchester Bombing, 15th June 1996, Actions and Lessons," *Fire Engineers Journal*, July 1997.

Borak, Jonathan, Michael Callan, and William Abbot. *Hazardous Materials Exposure*. Englewood Cliffs, NJ: Brady Publishers, 1991.

Bronstein, Alvin C., and Phillip L. Currance. *Emergency Care for Hazardous Materials Exposure*. St. Louis, MO: Mosby Year Book, 1994.

Buck, George. *Preparing for Terrorism: An Emergency Services Guide*. Albany, NY: Delmar Publishers, 1998.

Burdick, Brett A. (ed.). *Hazardous Materials Training/Public Safety Response to Terrorism (Student Manual)*. Richmond, VA: Virginia Department of Emergency Services, 1997.

Chemical/Biological Incident Handbook. Director of Central Intelligence, Interagency Intelligence Committee on Terrorism, Community Counterterrorism Board, June 1995.

Emergency Response to Terrorism: Incident Management (Student Manual). Emmitsburg, MD: U.S. Fire Administration/National Fire Academy, 1999.

Emergency Response to Terrorism: Job Aid. Emmitsburg, MD: U.S. Fire Administration/National Fire Academy, 2000.

Emergency Response to Terrorism: Self-Study. Emmitsburg, MD: U.S. Fire Administration/National Fire Academy, 1999.

Emergency Response to Terrorism: Tactical Considerations for Emergency Medical Services (Student Manual). Emmitsburg, MD: U.S. Fire Administration/National Fire Academy, 2000.

Marrs, Timothy C., Robert L. Maynard, and Fredrick R. Sidell. *Chemical Warfare Agents: Toxicology and Treatment*. Chichester, NY: Wiley, 1996.

Medical Management of Biological Casualties Handbook, 2nd Edition, U.S. Army Medical Research Institute of Infectious Diseases, 1996.

Medical Management of Chemical Casualties Handbook, 2nd Edition, U.S. Army Medical Research Institute of Chemical Defense, Chemical Casualty Care Office, 1995.

Medical Operations Considerations for WMD Incidents (Student Manual). St. Petersburg, FL: National Terrorism Preparedness Institute, 1998.

Medici, John, and Steve Patrick. *Emergency Response to Incidents Involving Chemical and Biological Warfare Agents*. Richmond, VA: Virginia Department of Emergency Services, 1996.

Noll, Gregory G., Michael S. Hildebrand, and James G. Yvorra. *Hazardous Materials: Managing the Incident*. International Fire Service Training Association, Fire Protection Publications, Oklahoma State University, 1994.

NIOSH Pocket Guide to Chemical Hazards. U.S. Department of Health and Human Services, Public Health Services, Centers for Disease Control, National Institute for Occupational Safety and Health, 2000.

North American Emergency Response Guidebook, U.S. Department of Transportation, Transport Canada, & Secretariat of Transport and Communications (Mexico). 2000.

Rhea, Steve. *Emergency Response to Bombing Incidents*. Richmond, VA: Virginia Department of Emergency Services, 1996.

Sachs, Gordon M. *Fire & EMS Department Safety Officer*. Englewood Cliffs, NJ: Brady Publishers, 2000.

Sachs, Gordon M. *Officer's Guide to Fire Service EMS*. Tulsa, OK: Pennwell, 1999.

Sidell, Frederick R. *Management of Chemical Warfare Agent Casualties*. Bel Air, MD: HB Publishing, 1995.

Sidell, Fredrick R., William C. Patrick, and Thomas Dashiell. *Jane's Chem-Bio Handbook*. Alexandria, VA: Jane's Information Group, 1998.

Smeby, Jr., L. Charles (ed.). *Hazardous Materials Response Handbook, 3rd Edition*. Quincy, MA: National Fire Protection Association, 1998.

Stilp, Richard, and Armando Bevelacqua. *Emergency Medical Response to Hazardous Materials Incidents*. Albany, NY: Delmar Publishers, 1997.

Stilp, Richard, and Armando Bevelacqua. *Hazardous Materials Field Guide*. Albany, NY: Delmar Publishers, 1998.

Stutz, Douglas R., and Scott Ulin. *Haztox, EMS Response to Hazardous Materials Incidents*. Miramar, FL: GDS Communications, 1993.

Wieder, Michael, Carol Smith, and Cynthia Brakhage (eds.). *Hazardous Materials for First Responders, 2nd Edition*. International Fire Service Training Association, Fire Protection Publications, Oklahoma State University, 1994.